GW00360433

SUPER FOOD

LEMON

B L O O M S B U R Y

LONDON · OXFORD · NEW YORK · NEW DELHI · SYDNEY

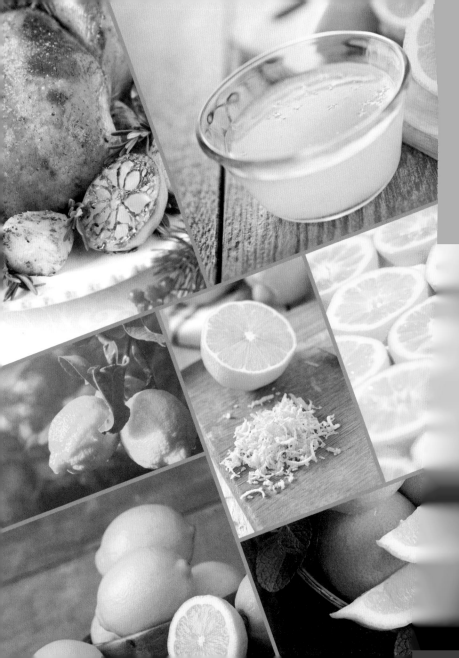

CONTENTS

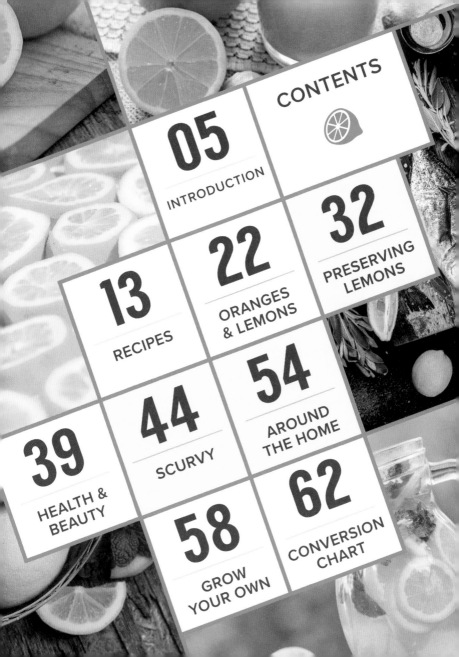

05 INTRODUCTION

13 RECIPES

22 ORANGES & LEMONS

32 PRESERVING LEMONS

39 HEALTH & BEAUTY

44 SCURVY

54 AROUND THE HOME

58 GROW YOUR OWN

62 CONVERSION CHART

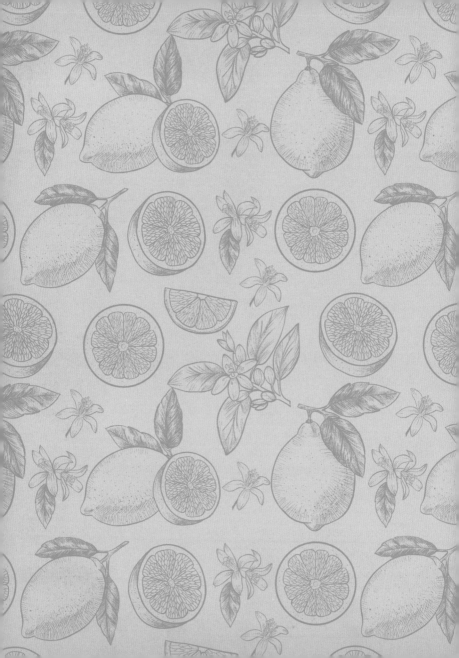

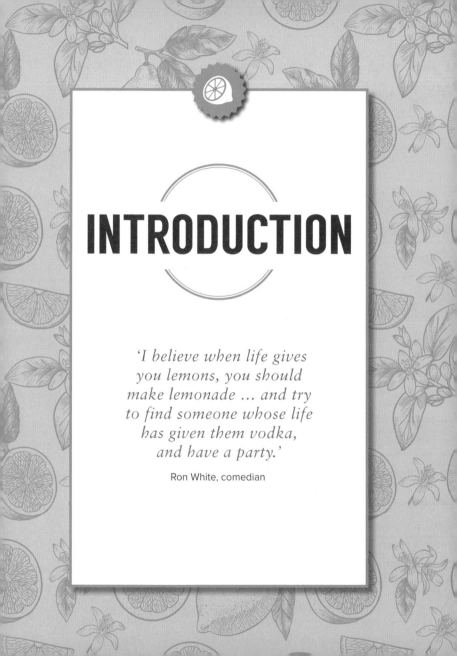

INTRODUCTION

'I believe when life gives
you lemons, you should
make lemonade ... and try
to find someone whose life
has given them vodka,
and have a party.'

Ron White, comedian

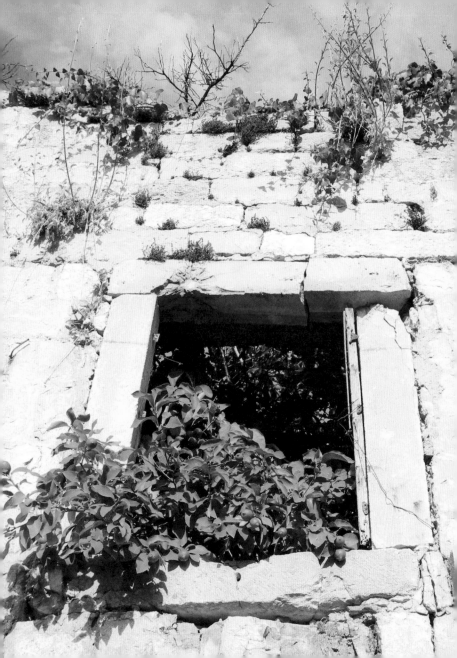

HISTORY

The first citrus trees grew millions of years ago, and it is thought that there were originally three varieties, mandarin, citron and pomelo, from which all modern citrus fruit, including lemons, derive.

The lemon is most closely related to the citron, which probably originated in the Punjab region of India and Pakistan, and from there spread via trading routes to the Middle East – excavations from Mesopotamia have revealed seeds dating to 4,000 BC. The citron travelled further west, arriving in the classical world probably by the 5th century BC, although it is difficult to trace its exact route. The word citron later came to refer to any type of citrus fruit, so references in ancient texts are ambiguous.

The Romans called the citron *malum medicum*. Virgil writes in the *Georgics* that the fruit came from Media (ancient Iran), and calls it the 'happy citron fruit', noting that it is used to chase 'black venom' from the body – an early recognition of its antiseptic properties. Indeed the ancient Romans used the citron primarily for medicinal purposes. It was believed that it cured all manner of complaints including snakebite, digestive problems and seasickness. The natural historian Pliny writes that the seeds were used as a breath freshener and it is said that the Emperor Nero consumed citrons to protect himself from poisoning attempts. The Greek philosopher and botanist Theophrastus wrote that the citron was not edible, but had an exquisite smell. The rind was used for flavouring, and the oil it contained was considered a luxury cosmetic, but the flesh was discarded as inedible.

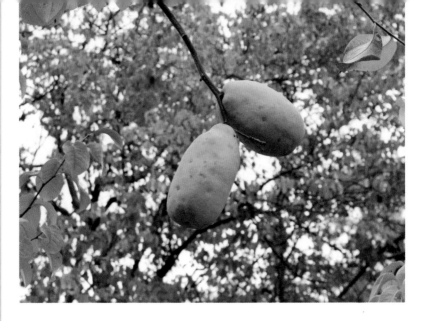

The modern lemon is thought to be a cross between the ancient citron and either a kind of sour orange or the mandarin. The earliest references to the modern form of lemon appear in Arabic writings of the 11th century AD. It is certain that the Arabs introduced the lemon to Europe in the 11th and 12th centuries. The Islamic world was enjoying a golden age at this time and was a major influence on Europe, with ideas in mathematics, art and science being adopted as well as new foodstuffs. The Crusaders bought lemons home to England with them from the Holy Land, and from the 14th century onwards they began to be a familiar item in well-to-do kitchens.

> *The Romans used the citron primarily for medicinal purposes.*

Lemons were being cultivated in Genoa, Italy, by the mid-15th century, and Columbus took lemon seeds with him on his second expedition to the New World in 1493, planting groves in Haiti and the Dominican Republic. The subsequent arrival of missionaries and explorers ensured the spread of the lemon throughout the Americas. As traders and colonisers crossed the globe during the 17th and 18th centuries the lemon went with them, particularly once it was used as a defence against scurvy. The First Fleet sent from Britain to Australia in 1787 took lemon trees with them for the new settlers to plant.

By the 19th century lemons were being imported into England from across Europe, and were also being grown in hothouses.

Once a luxury commodity, the lemon is now a familiar common and central part of our diet, and is appreciated for its taste as well as its health benefits in a wide range of recipes.

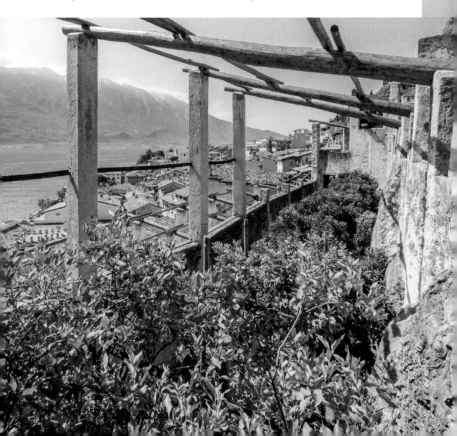

HEALTH BENEFITS

Lemons have been used in medicine for thousands of years as their health benefits have long been understood. The most well-known medicinal element of lemons is their high Vitamin C content, which has long made them a central ingredient in cold and flu remedies.

Vitamin C is an antioxidant, and lemons also contain flavonoids – together these fight infection and neutralise free radicals which cause disease and ageing.

The powerful antibacterial properties of lemons can destroy bacteria and purify the blood, thus helping to fight diseases such as malaria and cholera.

The citric acid is good for cleansing the digestive system – a glass of hot water with lemon in helps your liver flush away toxins more effectively, and improves bowel movements. It has also been suggested that lemon juice can dissolve kidney stones by removing the uric acid that causes them.

The lutein in lemons is good for preventing macular degeneration and cataracts in eyes, and promotes good skin. Eye and skin health and the immune system are also boosted by the presence of Vitamin A and rutin, which also helps regulate blood pressure.

Lemons contain several anti-carcinogenic compounds including limonene which has been shown to be highly effective in fighting cancer. Limonene has also been used in the treatment of gallstones.

Lemons contain a range of minerals including iron and copper, both essential for red blood cell production, to keep your body oxygenated. Other minerals include magnesium and

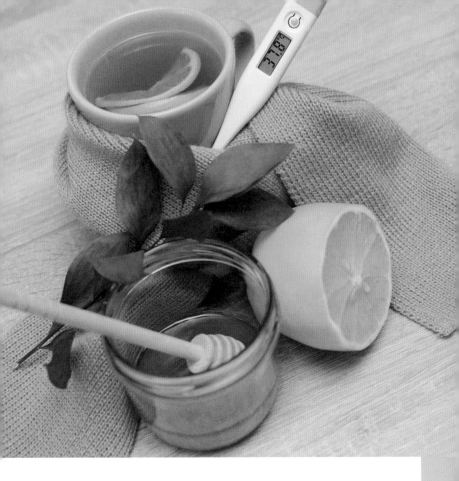

calcium which help with bone health. Potassium fights depression and aids digestion, and folate aids good heart health. Lemons are high in a healthy soluble fibre called pectin, which is good for lowering blood sugar.

Lemons are used in natural medicine for a huge range of treatments – for toothache, halitosis, soothing insect stings, for corns, and much more. There seems to be no end to the benefits of this mighty fruit!

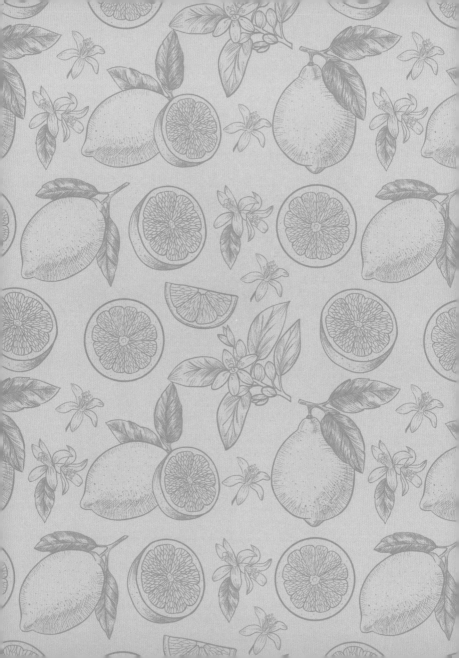

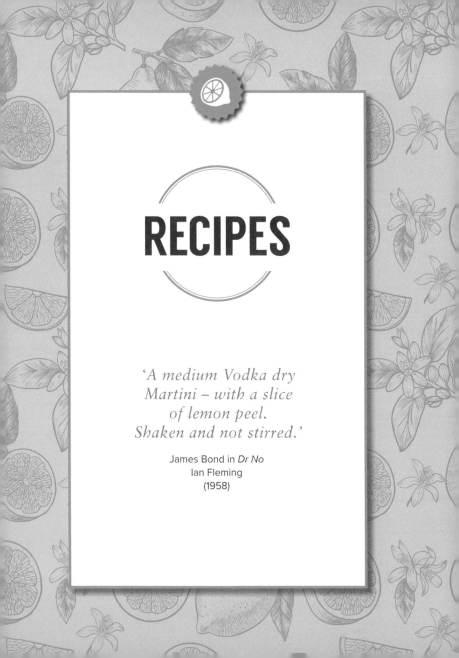

RECIPES

'A medium Vodka dry
Martini – with a slice
of lemon peel.
Shaken and not stirred.'

James Bond in *Dr No*
Ian Fleming
(1958)

SERVES: 2
PREPARATION: 5 MINUTES

BREAKFAST
SMOOTHIES

Drinking lemon juice is a great way to start your day – giving your system a Vitamin C boost and aiding digestion.

PEAR, BERRY & HONEY

The zesty lemon is sweetened with pear and honey in this smoothie bursting with antioxidants. Blend all the ingredients together, adding more honey if you need to.

INGREDIENTS

- juice of 1 lemon
- 1 pear, peeled and cored
- a handful of berries (you can use frozen ones)
- 2 tbsp honey
- 100ml water

BANANA, YOGHURT & CASHEW NUT

Yoghurt and banana are both excellent for digestion, and taste great with a burst of lemon added for freshness. Cashew nuts are packed with healthy nutrients.

INGREDIENTS

- juice of ½ lemon
- 1 banana
- 6 tbsp natural yoghurt
- 1 tbsp agave syrup
- a small a handful of cashew nuts

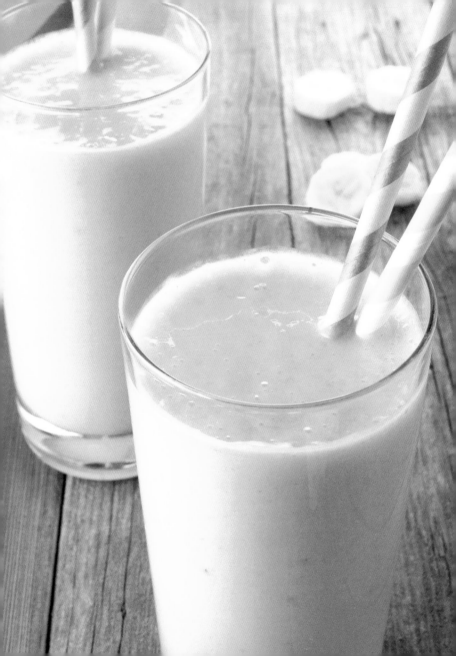

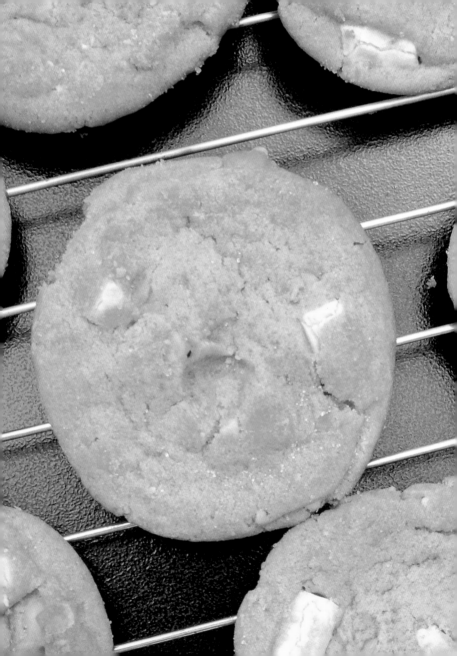

LEMON
BISCUITS

These delicious light biscuits are easy to make and even easier to eat! The white chocolate and lemon complement each other perfectly.

INGREDIENTS

- 125g butter
- 125g caster sugar
- yolk of 1 egg
- 170g self-raising flour
- zest of 1 lemon
- 100g white chocolate pieces

METHOD

Preheat oven to 180°C/350°F/gas mark 4.

Cream the butter and sugar and add the egg yolk. Sift in the flour and combine – you will get to the point where you need to use your hands to pull the mixture together. Grate the lemon zest into the mixture and add the chocolate pieces, kneading all together lightly.

Roll the biscuit dough out on a floured board and cut biscuit rounds with a cutter (or you can use the top of a glass). Place the biscuits on greased baking trays.

Bake for 15 minutes until light brown.

IN 1289 EDWARD I'S WIFE, ELEANOR OF CASTILE, HOMESICK FOR HER NATIVE LAND, SENT AN EMISSARY TO PORTSMOUTH TO BRING HER LEMONS FROM A SPANISH SHIP.

LEMON PASTA

Lemon juice adds a fresh lively twist to this creamy pasta dish with the subtle flavour of spinach and tangy Parmesan.

SERVES: 4
PREPARATION: 5 MINUTES
COOKING TIME: 15 MINUTES

INGREDIENTS

- 375g spaghetti
- juice of 2 lemons
- 50g butter
- 200ml double cream
- 200g spinach leaves
- 150g Parmesan cheese, grated
- salt and freshly ground black pepper

 TOP TIP

Why not add a handful of pine nuts for a variation?

METHOD

Cook the spaghetti according to the packet instructions. Meanwhile put the lemon juice, butter and cream into a small pan. Season to taste, bring to the boil and simmer until reduced.

When the pasta is nearly ready, add in the spinach leaves to wilt – this will only take a minute or so. Drain and add to the cream sauce with most of the Parmesan and toss together.

Serve with the remaining Parmesan grated over the top and plenty of freshly ground black pepper.

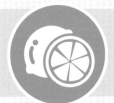

WHEN THE JEWS REVOLTED AGAINST THE ROMANS IN 66 AD THE LEMON WAS THE SYMBOL OF THEIR UPRISING.

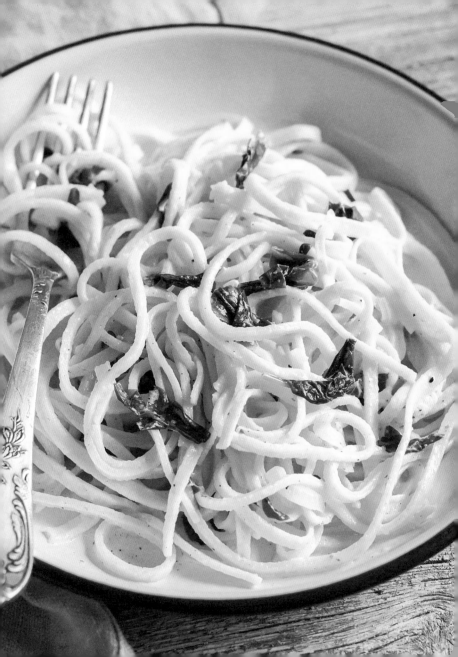

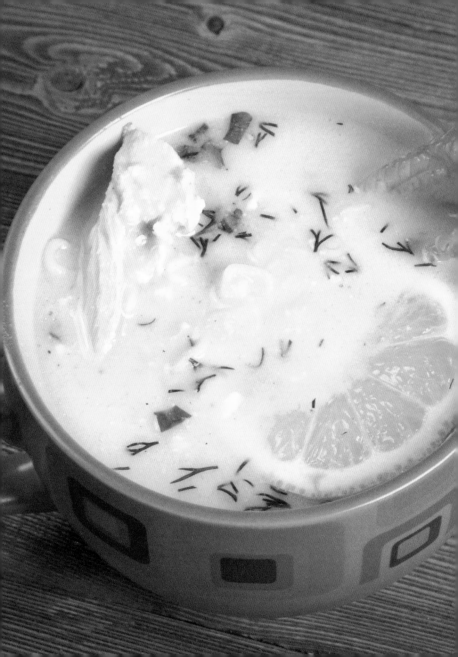

SERVES: 4
PREPARATION: 10 MINUTES
COOKING TIME: 15 MINUTES

AVGOLEMONO

Avgolemono is a traditional Greek soup, made with a sauce of eggs (*avgo*) and lemon (*lemono*). Nourishing and healthy, this soup reflects the Greek passion for the lemon in their cookery.

INGREDIENTS

- 1 tbsp olive oil
- 1 medium onion, chopped
- 2 cloves garlic, finely chopped
- 1 chicken breast, cut into strips
- 115g orzo pasta
- 1.75 litres chicken stock
- 3 eggs
- juice of 1 large lemon
- salt and freshly ground black pepper

METHOD

Heat the olive oil in a saucepan on a medium heat. Gently fry the onion and garlic until translucent, before adding the chicken strips and browning them for a few minutes.

Put the orzo into the pan and stir it around so it is fully coated in the flavours. Pour in the stock and bring to the boil, then simmer for 15 minutes until the orzo is soft and the chicken is cooked through. Remove the pan from the heat.

Beat the eggs well in a bowl, then whisk in the lemon juice and a tablespoon or so of cold water. Slowly stir in a ladleful of the cooled soup to the eggs, then add a couple more – going gently so the eggs don't curdle. Add the rest of the egg and lemon mixture to the saucepan, stirring all the time, and heat through very gently. Do not let the soup boil again!

Season to taste and serve.

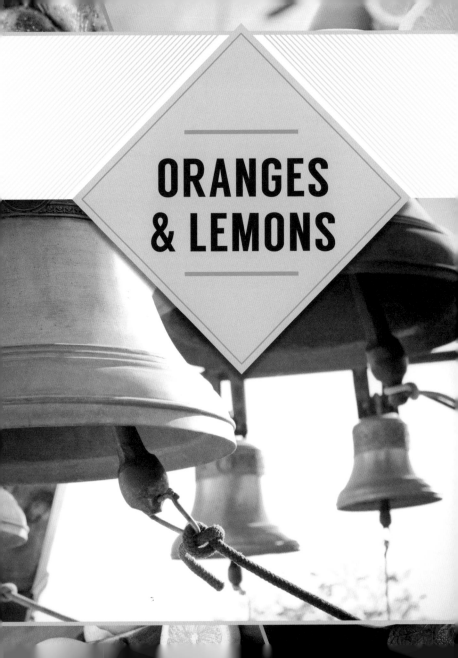

ORANGES & LEMONS

'Oranges and Lemons,'
say the bells of St Clement's.

'You owe me five farthings,'
say the bells of St Martin's.

'When will you pay me?'
say the bells of Old Bailey.

'When I grow rich,'
say the bells of Shoreditch.

'When will that be?'
say the bells of Stepney.

'I do not know,'
says the great bell of Bow.

The traditional nursery rhyme 'Oranges and Lemons' is one of the most famous of English rhymes, dating back hundreds of years, and listing many old churches in the City of London. 'The bells of St Clement's' are generally thought to mean those of St Clement's Church in Eastcheap and refer to the days when merchants landed shiploads of fruit at the nearby wharves. The bells were rung to mark the arrival of citrus fruits.

The church of St Clement Danes on the Strand, however, also lays claim to being the church of the rhyme, and its bells regularly ring out the well-known tune. In addition, children have annually celebrated an 'Oranges and Lemons Day' since 1919 when the church bells were re-hung. On 31st March each year children at the nearby St Clement Danes Church of England Primary School gather at the church to sing the nursery rhyme and to receive a gift of an orange and a lemon.

The rhyme was traditionally sung while children took part in a game or dance, which it is thought originated from a square dance for children entitled 'Oranges and Limons', included in a collection of dance music by John Playford dated 1651. (The first known printed version of 'Oranges and Lemons' appears to be in a work of around 1744 entitled *Tommy Thumb's Pretty Song Book*.)

While children sing the song two of them stand opposite each other holding hands and raising their arms in an arch while the other children run through. When they reach the final sinister line, 'Here comes the chopper to chop off your head' they lower the arch to catch the child going through at the time. In some versions the captured children then form more arches, but there are other ways to play.

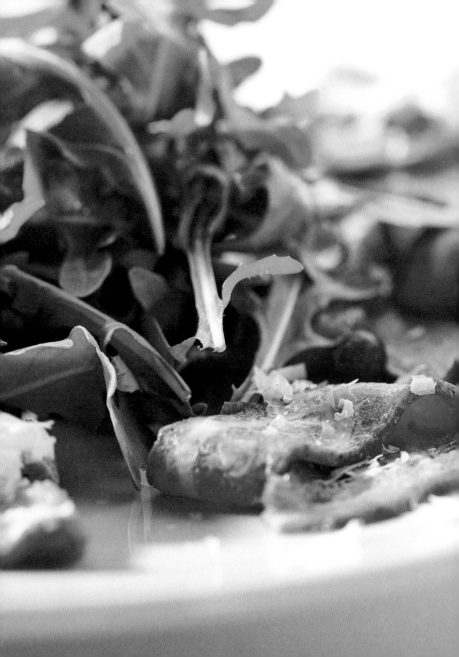

SERVES: 4
PREPARATION: 5 MINUTES

If you don't fancy raw meat, you can lightly sear the beef.

INGREDIENTS

- juice of 1½ lemons
- 50ml olive oil
- salt and freshly ground black pepper
- 4 very thin slices of the best quality fresh sirloin beef
- a handful of rocket leaves
- Parmesan, to garnish

CARPACCIO

The story goes that Carpaccio was invented in 1950 by Giuseppe Cipriani, chef at the famous Harry's bar in Venice. He based it on a Piedmontese dish and named it after his favourite artist, the 15th century Renaissance painter Vittore Carpaccio, whose use of vivid reds was evoked in the dish of raw meat.

METHOD

Whisk together the lemon juice and oil in a bowl, and season to taste.

Arrange the sliced beef on a plate and pour the dressing over the slices. Serve with fresh rocket leaves and Parmesan shavings.

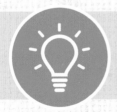

LEMONS GENERATE AN ELECTRICAL CURRENT WHEN THEIR ACID REACTS WITH METAL; HOWEVER IT WOULD TAKE THOUSANDS OF LEMONS TO POWER ONE LIGHT BULB.

SERVES: 4
PREPARATION: 10 MINUTES

 TOP TIP

You can try this dish with different types of fish – how about red snapper for something a bit different?

INGREDIENTS

- 500g halibut or monkfish
- 1 red onion, finely sliced
- 2 ripe tomatoes, chopped
- juice of 1 lemon
- juice of 1 lime
- 1 tbsp olive oil
- 1 green chilli, finely chopped
- 1 tsp oregano
- 1 tsp smoked paprika
- salt and freshly ground black pepper

CEVICHE

Ceviche is a popular dish from coastal Latin America, where raw fish is cured rather than cooked with heat, and spiced with garlic or chillies.

METHOD

Chop the fish into chunks and place in a shallow ceramic or glass dish with the red onion and tomatoes. In a small bowl mix together the lemon and lime juice, olive oil, chilli, oregano and paprika, and season to taste. Pour over the mixture in the dish, stirring well and making sure the fish is covered.

Cover and refrigerate for several hours, during which time you will see the fish change in colour as the acidic lemon and lime juices 'cook' it in the marinade.

Scatter the coriander leaves over the top to serve.

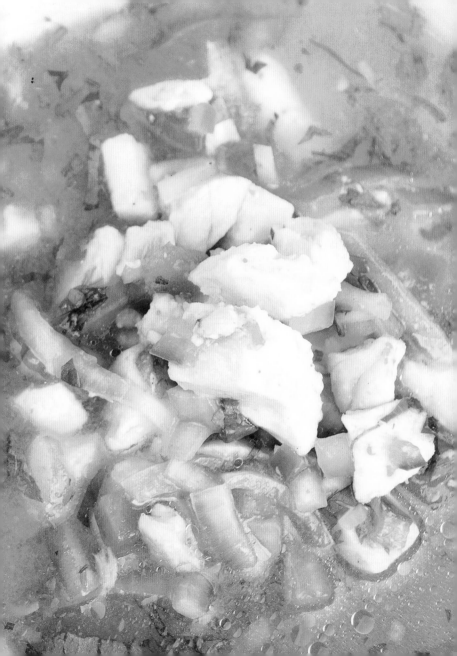

LEMON SOLE
WITH LEMON
& CAPERS

SERVES: **4**
PREPARATION: **10 MINUTES**
COOKING TIME: **4 MINUTES**

Lemon is perfect with any fish, and here the sharpness of the lemon is balanced by the sour saltiness of the capers in this quick and easy recipe. This light supper dish is delicious served with asparagus and new potatoes.

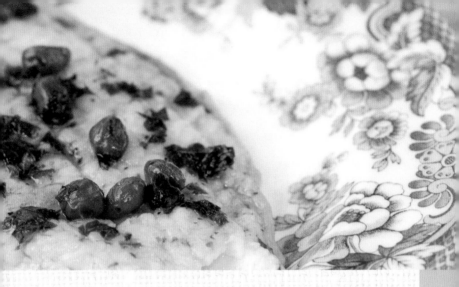

INGREDIENTS

- 60g butter
- 2 tbsp olive oil
- 4 lemon sole fillets
- 60ml lemon juice
- 30ml capers
- salt and freshly ground black pepper
- parsley to garnish
- lemon wedges, to serve

METHOD

Melt half of the butter with the olive oil in a heavy-based frying pan. Add the fish and fry it gently on each side for a couple of minutes, then take off the heat and keep warm on the serving plates.

Pour the lemon juice into the pan and melt the rest of the butter, before adding the capers and heating through. Pour the sauce over the fish and season. Serve with parsley garnish and lemon wedges.

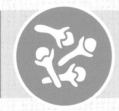

A LEMON STUCK WITH CLOVES WAS THOUGHT TO PURIFY THE AIR, AND IN A WORK OF 1636 WAS RECOMMENDED AS PROTECTION AGAINST THE PLAGUE.

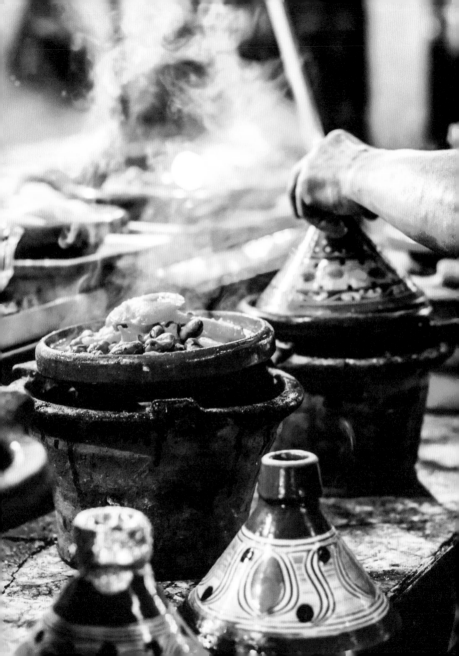

MOROCCAN TAGINE

SERVES: 4 – 6
PREPARATION: 15 MINUTES
COOKING TIME: 1 HR 30 MINUTES

Lemons and olives are classic components of Moroccan cuisine. Tagines are meat stews traditionally cooked by the nomadic Berbers in clay pots – you can use a casserole dish instead.

INGREDIENTS

- 2 tbsp olive oil
- 1 large onion
- 3 garlic cloves, crushed
- a thumb-sized piece of ginger, peeled and grated
- ½ tsp ground cinnamon
- pinch of saffron
- 4 chicken breasts on the bone
- 750ml chicken stock
- juice of 1 lemon
- a handful of coriander
- a handful of parsley
- 1 tsp coriander seeds
- 1 preserved lemon
- 115g green olives
- 1 tbsp honey
- salt and freshly ground black pepper

METHOD

Heat the olive oil in a casserole dish, chop the onion finely and sauté for five minutes or until translucent. Add the garlic to the pan with the ginger, cinnamon and saffron for a further minute.

Add the chicken breasts and cook until browned, turning them frequently. Finely chop the parsley and most of the coriander, reserving some leaves to garnish. Pour in the stock, lemon juice, herbs and coriander seeds and bring to the boil, then simmer for 45 minutes.

Rinse the preserved lemon in cold water, discard the flesh, and chop the peel. Stir into the pan with the olives and honey and simmer for 15 minutes.

Remove the chicken and keep it warm while you continue to heat the sauce until reduced. Pour the sauce over the chicken, season, and garnish with coriander and lemon slices.

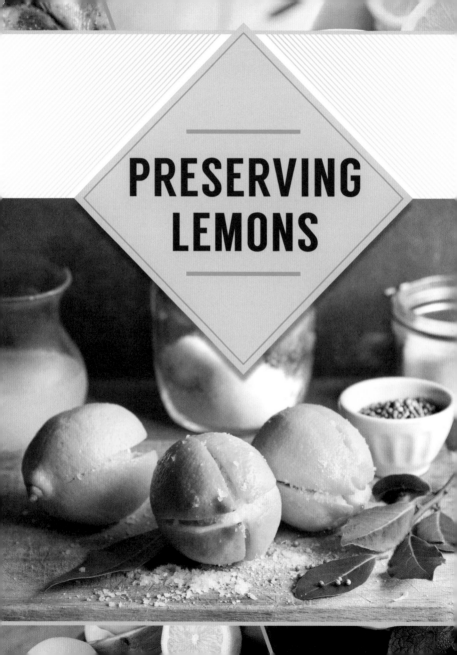

PRESERVING
LEMONS

Preserved lemons are a traditional ingredient in North African and Middle Eastern cuisine, adding a rich mellow flavour to dishes such as tagines and relishes.

Originally lemons were preserved in order to store them but preserved lemons are now appreciated for their unique taste.

It is simple to preserve lemons and you will find they will become an essential part of your store cupboard. They also make unusual and personal gifts, if you use really nice jars. Try them in dishes such as the Moroccan tagine on p 31.

METHOD

Sterilise the jar with boiling water, and wash the lemons thoroughly. Using a sharp knife, cut off the tips of the lemons at each end and then slice them into quarters, lengthwise, but stop before you completely detach the quarters, so they are attached along about 2cm at one end.

Cover the bottom of the jar with a layer of sea salt. Now sprinkle salt all over your lemon, spooning it inside

YOU WILL NEED:

- a glass jar
- approx 5 or 6 large organic lemons (for a ½ litre jar)
- sea salt, as needed
- olive oil, as needed

so the lemon is thoroughly coated inside and out.

Put the lemons in the jar, squashing each one down so the juices flow, and adding more salt as you go. Pack them down but leave a gap at the top of the jar, making sure they are submerged in juice. You may need to squeeze another lemon to make sure of this. Top up the mixture with salt and the olive oil. For an extra flavour, you could add a sprig of fresh thyme, or spices such as bay leaves or peppercorns.

Cover the jar and seal carefully. Store in a cool, dark place, and turn the jar upside down to shake the salt and juice around every couple of days for a week or so. After about three weeks the lemons will have softened and be ready for use. Rinse the salt from the lemon before using. They should keep for up to six months, if refrigerated.

MAKES: 4
PREPARATION: 2 HOURS
COOKING TIME: 20 MINUTES

LEMON MERINGUE PIE

The classic lemon pudding, a delicious mix of crumbly pastry, tangy lemon curd and light meringue.

INGREDIENTS

For the base:

- 215g shortcrust pastry

For the filling:

- 2 large egg yolks
- 30g caster sugar
- juice and zest of one lemon
- 30g white breadcrumbs
- 250ml milk

For the topping:

- 2 egg whites
- 115g caster sugar

METHOD

Roll out the pastry and line a pie dish. Chill the pastry for half an hour.

Put the egg yolks, sugar, lemon juice and zest and the breadcrumbs in a bowl, pour over the milk and mix well, before leaving for an hour until the breadcrumbs have absorbed the liquid.

Pre-heat oven to 190ºC/375ºF/gas mark 5.

Bake the pastry for ten minutes, using ceramic baking beans to prevent it rising in the oven. Turn the oven temperature down to 170ºC/325ºF/gas mark 3.

Mix the filling well and pour over the pastry, then return to the oven for five minutes to set the filling.

Whisk the egg whites until stiff, and gradually add the caster sugar, continuing to whisk until you have a glossy meringue. Heap the meringue on top of the lemon filling. Return to the oven for a further five minutes or until the meringue is a pale brown colour.

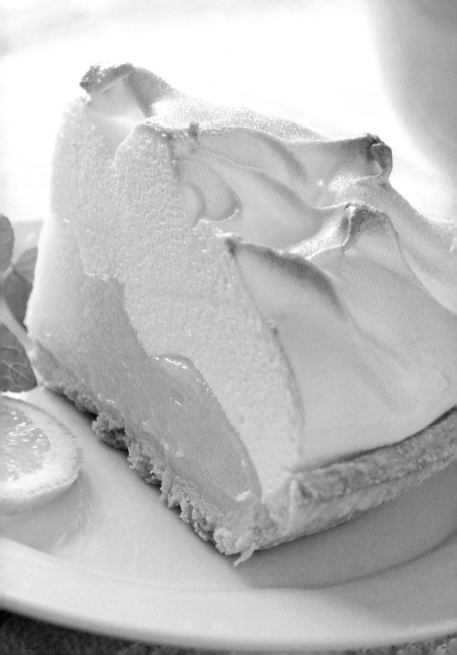

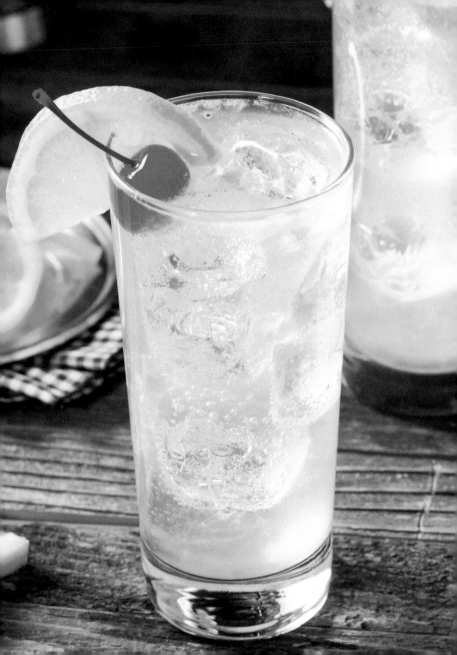

SERVES: 2
PREPARATION: 5 MINUTES

TOP TIP

Always use a highball glass, and if you can, frost it first by placing in the freezer for at least ten minutes.

INGREDIENTS

- a handful of ice cubes
- 60ml gin
- juice of ½ lemon
- 1 tbsp agave syrup
- soda water
- lemon wedge
- glacé cherry

TOM
COLLINS

The origin of the Tom Collins is disputed, but some claim it was created by a bartender, John Collins, at Limmer's Old House in Conduit Street, London, which was a popular sporting bar during the 19th century – famous for its 'gin-punch'.

METHOD

Pile a generous handful of ice cubes into your glass. Pour the gin and lemon juice over the ice, together with the agave syrup, and stir well.

Top with soda water and garnish with a lemon wedge and a glacé cherry!

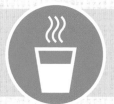

SIR EDMUND HILLARY DRANK COPIOUS QUANTITIES OF HOT WATER WITH LEMON DURING HIS ASCENT OF EVEREST IN 1953.

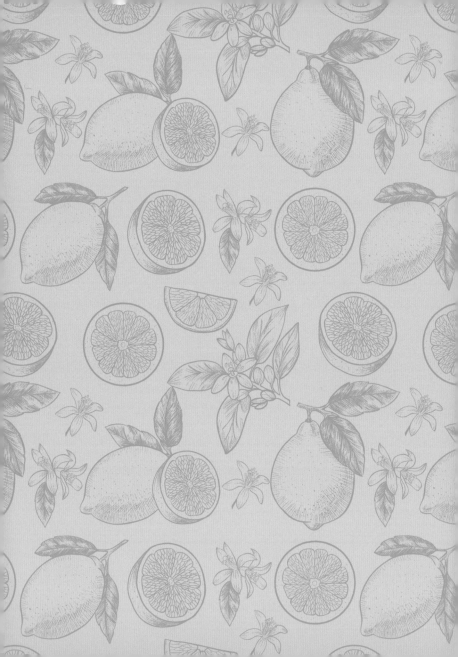

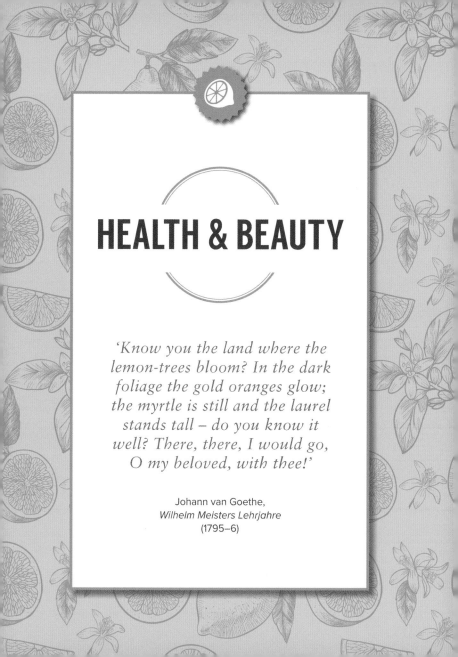

HEALTH & BEAUTY

'Know you the land where the lemon-trees bloom? In the dark foliage the gold oranges glow; the myrtle is still and the laurel stands tall – do you know it well? There, there, I would go, O my beloved, with thee!'

Johann van Goethe,
Wilhelm Meisters Lehrjahre
(1795–6)

TURMERIC AND GREEN TEA MASK

 TOP TIP

For extra acne-fighting properties, add one whisked egg white. The egg reduces pore size, reduces sebum production and also maintains a healthy Ph balance for your skin.

This powerful combination of ingredients forms an amazing, multi-tasking mask. Not only does it provide natural antioxidant protection and skin-nourishing vitamins, but it kills skin bacteria, fights fine lines and wrinkles, has anti-inflammatory properties, can lighten pigmentation and even protect your skin from harmful UV rays. What more could you ask for from a mask?!

INGREDIENTS

- 3 tbsp cooled green tea
- a small pinch of turmeric
- 1 tsp lemon juice

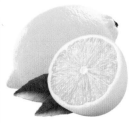

METHOD

Combine the ingredients in a bowl.

Exfoliate your skin to allow for maximum penetration of the mask. Dampen but don't saturate a cotton wool pad with the liquid.

Sweep over your face to leave a thin layer and allow to dry for a few minutes. When dry repeat the process until most or all of the mixture is used up.

Relax for 20 minutes before gently rinsing off.

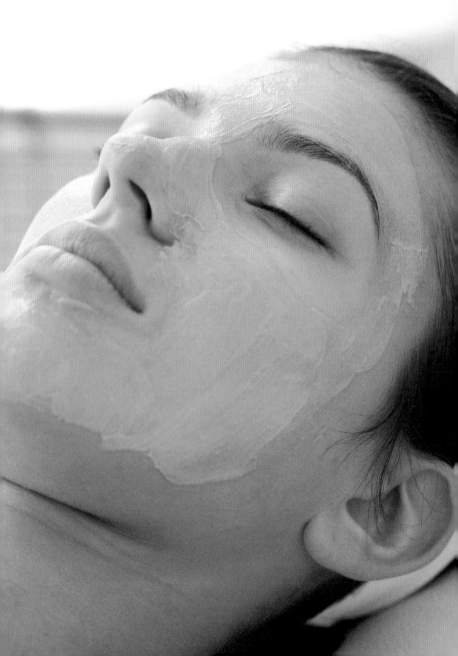

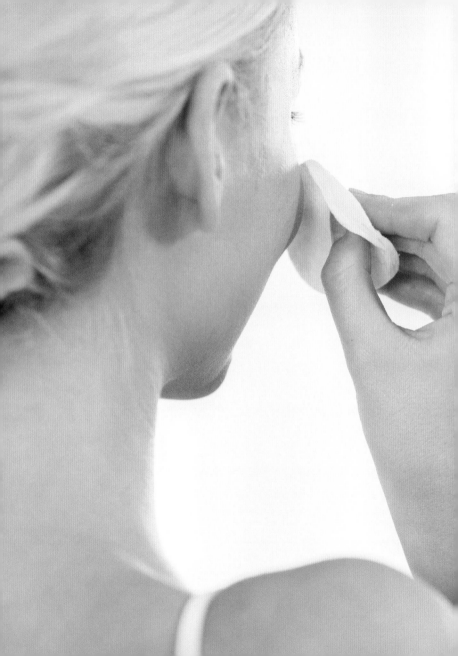

WITCH HAZEL, CUCUMBER & GREEN TEA TONER

This super refreshing toner is so lovely to use, and so simple to make, you'll never go back to buying an off-the-shelf toner again!

METHOD

Blitz the ingredients together in a blender until the cucumber becomes a fine pulp. Strain it through cheesecloth and reserve the liquid. Pour it into a clean, sterile bottle, making sure you squeeze every drop of juice from the pulp, too.

Pour a 10p-sized amount onto a cotton wool pad and sweep over your face after cleansing. You can keep the toner for a few weeks, but be sure to store in the fridge between uses.

INGREDIENTS

- ½ peeled cucumber
- juice of ½ lemon
- 100ml witch hazel
- 80ml cooled green tea

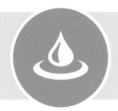

APPLYING LEMON JUICE DIRECT TO SPOTS AND ACNE CAN HELP FIGHT THE BACTERIA THAT CAUSES THEM.

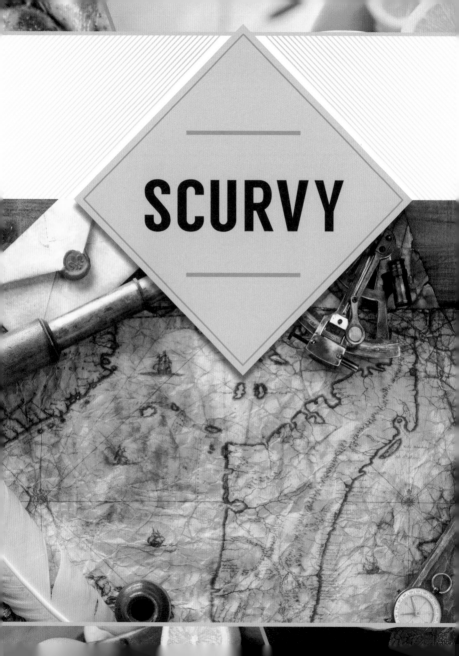

SCURVY

Scurvy – the word comes from the Latin word *scorbotus* – has been plaguing humans since ancient times.

It is a disease caused by a lack of Vitamin C and has a range of unpleasant symptoms including fever, swelling limbs, bleeding and paralysis.

During the 16th to 18th centuries scurvy became particularly associated with sailors who sailed great distances without sufficient fresh foods. For sailors, it was a greater threat than enemy action, and during one expedition alone in the 1740s nearly three-quarters of the crew were lost to illness. It was a huge problem, as the naval surgeon James Lind noted, 'the scurvy alone, during the last war, proved a more destructive enemy, and cut off more valuable lives, than the united efforts of the French and Spanish arms.'

The benefits of citrus fruits to combat scurvy had been recognised early, but provisions on board did not regularly include them. Admiral Richard Hawkins had realised in the 16th century that scurvy could be defeated by serving the sailors three spoonfuls of lemon juice each day. He wrote that the best remedy was the use of 'sour oranges and lemons'.

In a 1636 work on Naval Surgery it was noted that 'The use of the juice of lemons is a precious medicine, and well tried; being sound and good, let it have the chief place, for it will deserve it; the use whereof is: It is to be taken each morning, two or three spoonfuls ... .' But although this knowledge was available, it was still not properly understood, and expeditions that followed failed to take the advice, more generally attempting other remedies such as

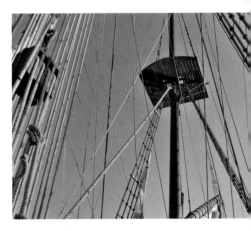

blood-letting, elixir of vitriol and countering the bad effect of sea air by putting turf on the patient's mouth!

In 1747 James Lind was the surgeon aboard HMS *Salisbury* when there was a serious outbreak of scurvy. He carried out what became the first controlled experiment to try and tackle scurvy. He had 12 patients whose symptoms were 'as similar as I could have them. They all in general had putrid gums, the spots and lassitude, with weakness of their knees.' He gave them all the same diet but divided them into six groups on whom he tested different remedies, including one group who received two oranges and one lemon each day. 'The consequence was, that the most sudden and visible good effects were perceived from the use of the oranges and lemons ... .' By the end of the week's trial those men were better.

Unfortunately these results did not attract much attention, and James Lind left the navy and returned to practice in Edinburgh. Although he published a book, *A Treatise of the Scurvy*, in which he detailed his experiment, he deduced that scurvy was a result of cold moist air and only partly caused by diet, and thus left no clear conclusion explaining the connection between Vitamin C and scurvy. He died in 1794.

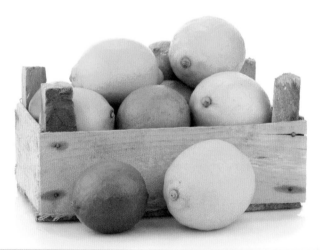

Sir Gilbert Blane had been appointed as physician to the British fleet in 1780, and at his suggestion, an experiment carried out in 1795 proved Lind's theory again. A ship, the *Suffolk*, left England and arrived in Madras 162 days later with no sickness, after each man was issued ⅔ oz lemon juice and 2 oz sugar mixed in with his daily grog. 'She lost not a man; and though the disease

> *The benefits of citrus fruits to combat scurvy had been recognised early, but provisions on board did not regularly include them.*

made its appearance in a few, an increased dose of lemon-juice immediately removed it.' Another ship, the *Centurion*, made a similar length journey and lost half her crew.

The Scottish naval physician Thomas Trotter had also corroborated Lind's thesis by his own observations and shared his belief in the advocacy of lemon juice, firing off a series of missives to the Admiralty. He vented his frustration at the lack of progress, especially after the disaster of the *Centurion* in 1795:

'The lemon, and all fruits of that class, have been known as effective cures for scurvy for more than 200 years. But so defective were the arrangements in the medical department, that not a single chest of lemons or oranges were ever seen in store, or on a king's shop, on home service, where the disease was most apt to appear in its hideous forms.' (*Monthly Magazine*, 1822)

Finally, in 1795, the year after James Lind's death, at Blane's insistence, 75 oz per day of lemon juice became standard issue in the British Navy. Within 50 years scurvy had been eliminated, although it reappeared in the late 19th century after lime juice was substituted for the lemon juice. Limes, which gave the sailors their nicknames of 'Limeys', have an ascorbic acid rate of one-third less than lemons and oranges.

Today, James Lind is honoured by the Institute of Naval Medicine as the father of naval medicine. The official crest of the Institute features a lemon tree, and the British Navy requires all ships to carry enough lemons so that every sailor can have an ounce of juice a day.

LEMON & PEPPERMINT FOOT SCRUB

Give your feet a treat with this divinely-scented, refreshing foot scrub. It's so quick and easy to make and use, and you'll immediately see and feel the results! You'll need a clean, sterilised jam jar as this can be kept and re-used.

INGREDIENTS

- 250g sea salt
- 2 tbsp nut oil (almond is best)
- 3 tsp lemon zest and a few drops of juice
- 10 drops peppermint oil

METHOD .

Simply mix the ingredients together and store in a jam jar. Keep it in the fridge between uses.

Soak your feet for a few minutes in warm water, then take a scoop of salt scrub and gently massage all over your feet for a few minutes. Pay extra attention to areas with harder skin such as your heels.

Rinse off and ideally follow with a moisturising lotion to enjoy baby-soft feet for days!

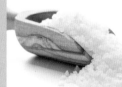

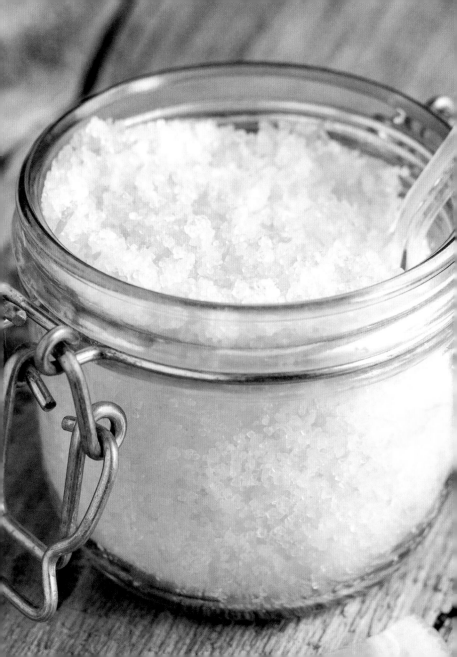

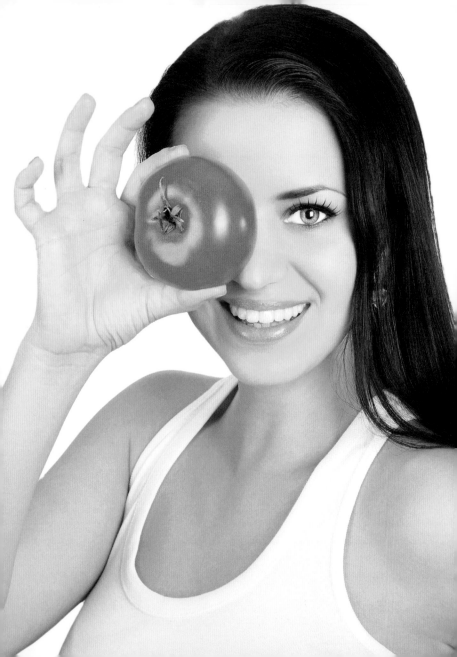

LEMON & TOMATO EYE TREATMENT

Tomato and lemon creates a powerful combination to help fight dark circles and regenerate puffy, tired skin around the eye area. This mask is packed with Vitamins A and B, great for skin renewal and cell turnover, and is so simple to make and use!

METHOD

Simply combine the juices and sweep over the under eye area. Be very careful not to get the juice in your eyes. If you do, wash immediately with cold water.

Leave the mixture on for 30–40 minutes and rinse. Also be careful when rinsing off not to splash the treatment into your eyes.

INGREDIENTS

- juice of 1 lemon
- juice of 1 tomato

 TOP TIP

Try to use best quality locally-sourced tomatoes as supermarket ones suffer during tranportation and storage and can contain less nutrients.

COCONUT & LEMON DAMAGE REPAIR MASK

Lemon juice has multiple benefits for hair and scalp. It can treat dandruff, itchy scalp, stimulate hair growth and even help to straighten and tame unruly frizz.

INGREDIENTS

- 60ml lemon juice
- 200g coconut oil

TOP TIP

To tackle dandruff you can apply lemon juice direct to your scalp and massage for around 20 minutes before rinsing out.

METHOD

Mix the lemon juice and coconut oil together until completely blended.

Use a comb or your fingers to coat your hair and scalp with the mixture and be sure to work it right through to the ends.

Wrap your hair in a warm towel or in clingfilm and leave the mask to work its magic for around 20 minutes.

If you can do this while relaxing in the bath, the heat and steam will help the mask to work even more effectively.

Wash out thoroughly for beautiful, shiny, manageable hair.

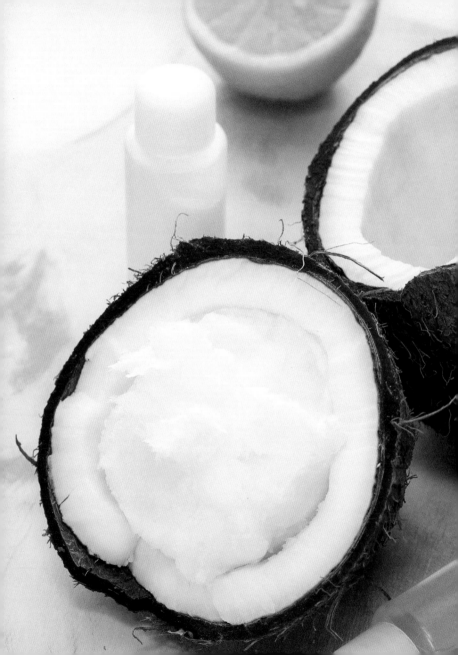

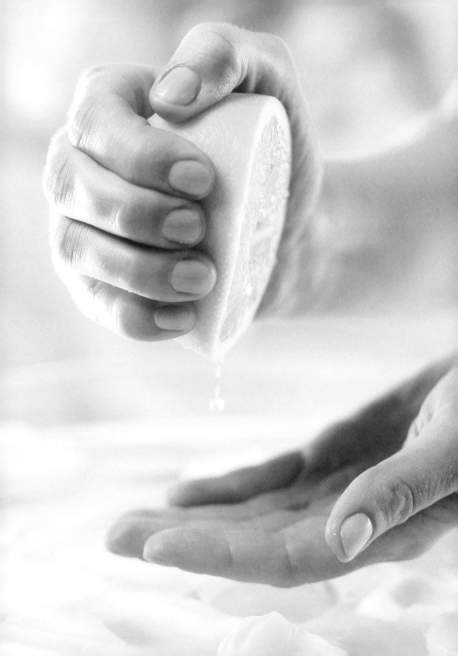

NAIL STRENGTHENER

Broken, chipped nails are an aggravating, but totally avoidable problem. The issue with nails is almost always lack of moisture and this leads to brittleness and weakness in the nail. Before you rush out and spend a fortune on shop-bought chemical products, here's a simple and highly effective treatment you can make yourself.

METHOD

Combine the lemon juice and olive oil in a small bowl with the essential oil if using. Warm the mixture in a small pan on a very gentle heat, or in a microwave for a few seconds. When the mixture is cool, pour into a clean, sterile bottle.

Apply a generous amount to a cotton pad and coat the whole of each nail and surrounding area with the treatment.

You can repeat this treatment as often as you like!

YOU WILL NEED

- 3 tbsp olive oil
- 1 tbsp lemon juice
- 2 drops lavender oil (optional)

 TOP TIP

Apply at bedtime and wear some cotton manicure gloves for an extra intensive and luxurious treatment.

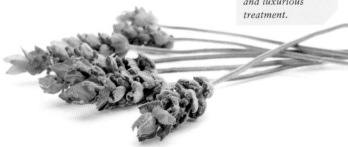

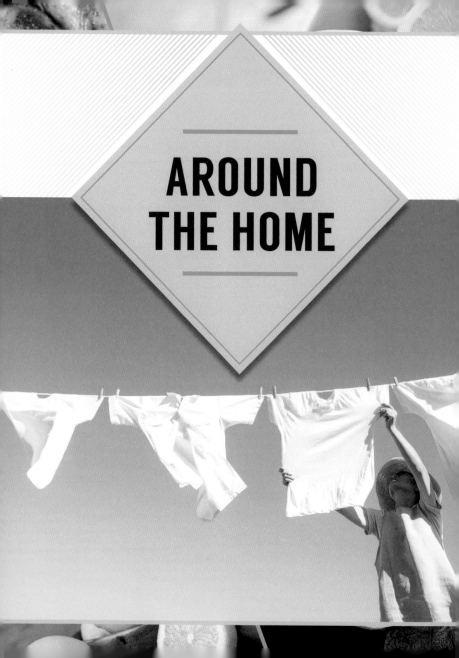

AROUND THE HOME

Lemons can be used in many ways around the home, due to the antibacterial properties of the juice and the natural oils in the peel – here are a few ideas.

LAUNDRY

Adding a teaspoon of lemon juice to your wash can make your clothes smell fresher and your whites whiter, while lemon juice can be used to remove stains. Let the juice dry on the stain before washing out.

MOTHS

Dried lemon peel can be hung in your cupboards to keep moths at bay and protect your clothes, for a chemical-free solution to an age-old problem.

FIRELIGHTERS

The natural oils in lemon peel make them good to use as firelighters. Dry the peels out in the oven at a low temperature until they harden.

CLEANING

Remove stains from chopping boards and freshen them up by rubbing them with lemon juice. You can also use lemons as a limescale remover. Cut a lemon up and place it on limescale stains for an hour, then scrub off.

MIRRORS

You can also clean mirrors by adding the juice of half a lemon to 4 litres of water and wiping the mirror with a cloth. Or you can simply apply the juice directly to any stubborn stains.

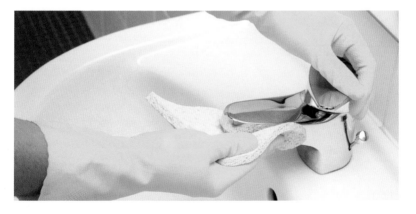

GROW YOUR OWN

You can grow a lemon tree from seed although often they are propagated by rooting cuttings.

To grow from seed you will need to buy an organic lemon as these are more likely to have seeds that will germinate. Extract the seeds and remove all the pulp. Be ready to plant your seed immediately before it dries out.

Fill a pot with some good quality potting compost, with vermiculite included to aid drainage. Water the soil first and mix the water through so that the soil is moist but not too saturated.

Plant your seed at a depth of around 2cm and cover with soil. Cover the pot with clingfilm or a clear plastic bag and make sure the edges are sealed – you can use a rubber band. Poke a few holes in the plastic and set the pot in a warm, sunny place.

Make sure the soil does not dry out over the next couple of weeks while you wait for the seed to germinate. Once the seedling appears, remove the cover. Keep watering your seedling and keep it in a light place – you may want to use a grow light if you are keeping it indoors. Feed it with a good-quality nitrogen-rich plant food.

Once the plant reaches around 30cm high you will need to repot it, making sure the soil remains damp and well drained.

Lemon trees need to be kept warm so if you are going to have your pot in the garden you will need to bring it inside during the winter months.

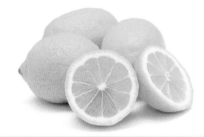

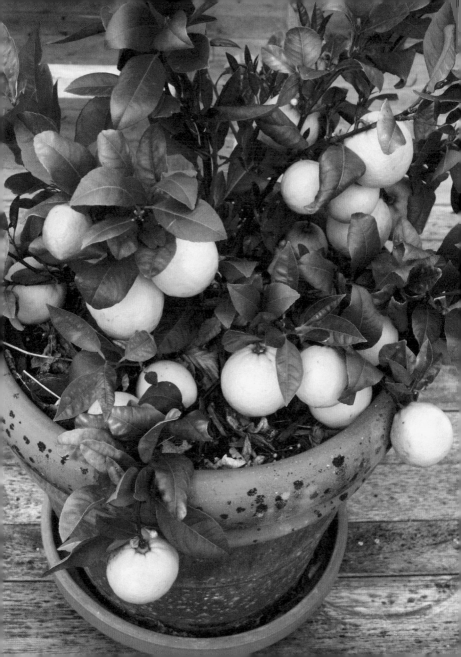

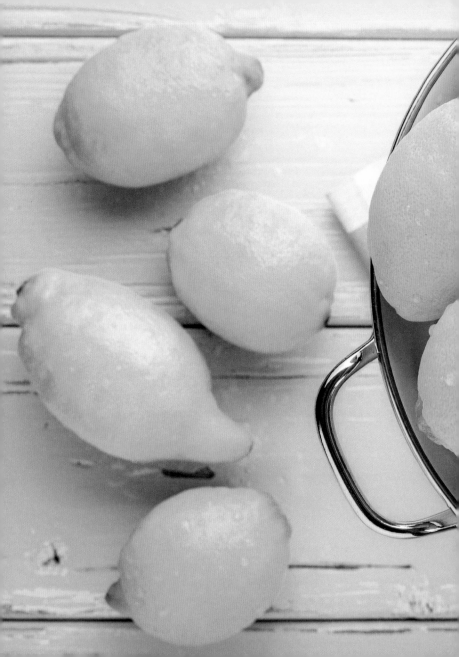

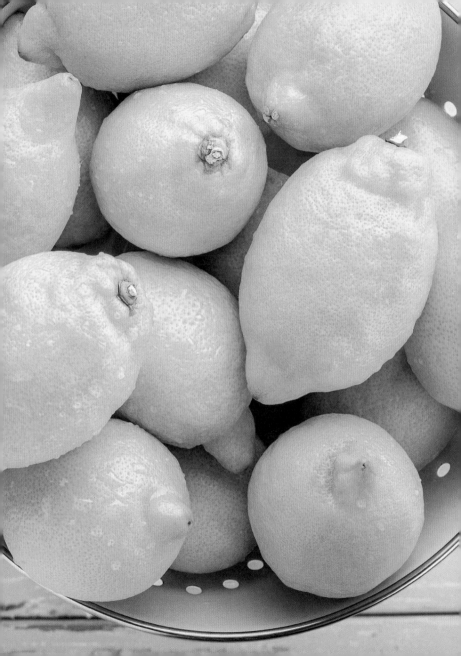

CONVERSION CHART
FOR COMMON MEASUREMENTS

LIQUIDS

15 ml	½ fl oz
25 ml	1 fl oz
50 ml	2 fl oz
75 ml	3 fl oz
100 ml	3 ½ fl oz
125 ml	4 fl oz
150 ml	¼ pint
175 ml	6 fl oz
200 ml	7 fl oz
250 ml	8 fl oz
275 ml	9 fl oz
300 ml	½ pint
325 ml	11 fl oz
350 ml	12 fl oz
375 ml	13 fl oz
400 ml	14 fl oz
450 ml	¾ pint
475 ml	16 fl oz
500 ml	17 fl oz
575 ml	18 fl oz
600 ml	1 pint
750 ml	1 ¼ pints
900 ml	1 ½ pints
1 litre	1 ¾ pints
1.2 litres	2 pints
1.5 litres	2 ½ pints
1.8 litres	3 pints
2 litres	3 ½ pints
2.5 litres	4 pints
3.6 litres	6 pints

WEIGHTS

5 g	¼ oz
15 g	½ oz
20 g	¾ oz
25 g	1 oz
50 g	2 oz
75 g	3 oz
125 g	4 oz
150 g	5 oz
175 g	6 oz
200 g	7 oz
250 g	8 oz
275 g	9 oz
300 g	10 oz
325 g	11 oz
375 g	12 oz
400 g	13 oz
425 g	14 oz
475 g	15 oz
500 g	1 lb
625 g	1 ¼ lb
750 g	1 ½ lb
875 g	1 ¾ lb
1 kg	2 lb
1.25 kg	2 ½ lb
1.5 kg	3 lb
1.75 kg	3 ½ lb
2 kg	4 lb

OVEN TEMPERATURES

110°C .... (225°F) .... gas mark ¼
120°C .... (250°F) .... gas mark ½
140°C .... (275°F) .... gas mark 1
150°C .... (300°F) .... gas mark 2
160°C .... (325°F) .... gas mark 3
180°C .... (350°F) .... gas mark 4
190°C .... (375°F) .... gas mark 5
200°C .... (400°F) .... gas mark 6
220°C .... (425°F) .... gas mark 7
230°C .... (450°F) .... gas mark 8

MEASUREMENTS

5 mm .... ¼ inch
1 cm .... ½ inch
1.5 cm .... ¾ inch
2.5 cm .... 1 inch
5 cm .... 2 inches
7 cm .... 3 inches
10 cm .... 4 inches
12 cm .... 5 inches
15 cm .... 6 inches
18 cm .... 7 inches
20 cm .... 8 inches
23 cm .... 9 inches
25 cm .... 10 inches
28 cm .... 11 inches
30 cm .... 12 inches
33 cm .... 13 inches

KEY TO SYMBOLS

(DF) Dairy free

(GF) Gluten free

(V) Vegetarian

(VG) Vegan

A NOTE ON USING DIFFERENT OVENS

Not all ovens are the same, and the more cooking you do the better you will get to know yours. If a recipe says that you need to bake something for ten minutes or until golden brown, use your judgment as to whether it needs a few extra minutes. Conversely don't overcook food by following the timings rigidly if you think it looks ready.

As a general rule gas ovens have more uneven heat distribution so the top of the oven may be hotter than the bottom. Electric ovens tend to maintain a regular temperature throughout and distribute heat more evenly, especially fan ovens.

All the recipes in this book have been tested in an electric oven with a fan. Recommended oven temperatures are provided for electric (Celsius and Fahrenheit), and gas. If you have a fan oven then lower the electric temperature by 20°.

Bloomsbury Publishing
An imprint of Bloomsbury Publishing plc

50 Bedford Square
London
WC1B 3DP
UK

1385 Broadway
New York
NY 10018
USA

www.bloomsbury.com

BLOOMSBURY and the Diana logo are trademarks of Bloomsbury Publishing Plc

First Published in 2017

© Bloomsbury Publishing plc

Created for Bloomsbury by Plum5 Ltd

Photographs and Illustrations © Shutterstock

British Library Cataloguing-in-Publication Data

A catalogue record for this book is available from the British Library.

Library of Congress Cataloguing-in-Publication Data

A catalogue record for this book is available from the Library of Congress.

ISBN: 9781408887288

2 4 6 8 10 9 7 5 3 1

Printed in China by C&C Printing

To find out more about our authors and books visit www.bloomsbury.com.
Here you will find extracts, author interviews, details of forthcoming events
and the option to sign up for our newsletters.